MASTERING PEST CONTROL: Expert Tips and Techniques to Keep Your Space Bug-Free

Natalie Luis

Table of Contents

CHAPTER ONE

INTRODUCTION

Bug control will be a basic gamble for mankind in the approaching future. Eventually we will be overall impacted by aggravates as it is admirably present all over. Whether it is bugs or scarabs in the kitchen or weeds in the vegetable nursery, aggravations can agitate. Simultaneously, huge amounts of us are not roused by bug control and the issues accomplished by disturbs as well as the pesticides we use to control bugs. Bugs are useful as well as a reprimand to mankind. Creatures, microorganisms and two or three bugs are valuable to individuals in different ways, yet similar time they can likewise be aggravations. Vermin, for example, rodents, underground bugs, cockroaches, mice and flies are normal in houses and lofts. There ought to be a persuading unsettling influence control to impede bugs in duplicating themselves in houses, which merge sensible irritating the board, bug control and vermin avoidance.

BUG THE BOSSES

The unendingly best way for controlling unsettling influences is vermin the board which coordinates many advances. The first and most immense stage in Vermin Control is to perceive the bug issue. This combines sorting out unequivocally exact thing you are going up against. Two or three aggravations (microorganisms, creatures) are truly useful to individuals, so figuring out any hazardous vermin is essential. The subsequent thing is to wrap up how much vermin control is focal. Basically the family who live in the impacted region can presume that making a move is so serious. The third thing is to pick an open choice for inconvenience control, for example, substance bug control or non produced bug control. You have some control over bugs by various strategies; a piece of the choices open are:

Non Compound disturbance control

Designed bug control

Customary Strategies

One more remarkable answer for bug control is the utilization of fabricated pesticides. It isn't wise in and around the home and business premises, as it will affect individuals horrendously. The enormous shortcoming of this methodology is the inevitable result of the designed pesticides treatment which is for the most part short, which hence need emphasized prescriptions. Whenever utilized mistakenly, home-use pesticides can be harmful to people. While you are including compound pesticides for bug control, the primary concern to recall is to take care in picking the right pesticide thing. One more sensible way in controlling vermin is utilizing the ordinary technique. This is the strategy for utilizing disturbance's common adversaries to control them. Bugs, centipedes, ground upsetting little animals and bugs are a piece of the valuable bugs. This system isn't unsafe to individuals in any means and can be finished really.

DIY HOME VERMIN CONTROL

Basically all property holders would feel horrendous tolerating they observed that bugs are accumulating their homes. Close by wrecking your property, they can likewise cause clinical issues for yourself as well as your loved ones. Killing them ought to be your need and most frequently, applying DIY structure works wonder. Precisely when bug issues have caused tremendous harms, bug control associations might be indispensable. At last, tolerating you are basically doing some preventive assistance, DIY can assist you with scarcely scraping by. The chief concern is frustrating vermin in your house is focal both for your property and for your family as well. A colossal piece of us got past difficulty gives that need serious areas of strength for an arrangement. Doing your own bug the bosses has been reasonable in directing bug issues in nursery, homes, and business as well. Utilizing sensible things and supplies will empower you to dispose of aggravations in confinement, without looking for skilled assistance from inconvenience the board affiliations and pay for their costly associations and remedies. Various individuals have been gotten the hang of concerning managing vermin issues. DIY bug control things and supplies are turning out to be huge for each family's requirements. Whether you truly need to kill bugs, termites, underground bugs, or kissing bugs, top of the line DIY inconvenience control pesticides and things will give you the best outcome that you really want for your home, property and family's security. Close to being reasonable, DIY inconvenience controls will make you set aside cash without giving up the possibility of the things and its appropriateness. It will give you the best vermin course of action the same way that experts outfit you with their association just significantly more reasonable. Things for rodents and bugs are additionally open for family and business use. Do-It-Yourself inconvenience control things are open in commonplace and ordinary strategy.

Do-It-Yourself things can truly set aside you money than purchasing costly brands with practically identical decorations and definition. They have various things like sprinkles, gets, dust, spread, shadiness, and fog for frustrating different sorts of bugs. You should simply figure out the proper thing for your requirements and you can right now manage your nervousness secluded. Specialists for DIY inconvenience controls can assist you with finding the correct thing by offering you the best thing answer for your aggravation issues. Do-It-Yourself bug things are exceptional both in regulating aggravations outside like flies and mosquitoes and indoor vermin like cockroaches, rodents, bugs, termites and different others. Undoubtedly, even without skilled assistance, you will figure out that vermin control is clear as well as making your home disturbance free. Preventive measures are critical in keeping aggravation free homes. Inconvenience control supplies are comparably useful in doing the preventive measures. Reliably survey that annoying control doesn't ensure everything. There might be two or three Do-It-Yourself methodologies and things that may just fight bugs off immediately and a brief time frame later they will return. In cases like these, Do-It-

Yourself could dial back you more than looking for proficient assistance. It is no question that fit bug control associations has high customer endurance rating. For you to be sensible in your Do-It-Yourself program, ensure that you essentially utilize productive things and pesticides since there are different lacking pesticides out there. Furthermore, to make it more useful, you can introduce demands from Do-It-Yourself prepared experts and they will merrily add information in you. Coming up next are several genuine variables and aggravation control things that are effectively open in the house:

Garlic. This is a brand name bug repellant and a trademark pesticide for your nursery.

Spreading out garlic close by tomatoes can frustrate red bug parasites.

Applying garlic sprinkle on making potatoes can ward hares off.

Showering garlic pesticides on water bowls and lakes will kill mosquitoes.

Onions and mint are really ideally suited for loathsome little animals, endlessly messes with.

Borax or boric disastrous is ideal in getting out cockroaches, ticks, bugs, termites, bugs, and some more. It additionally abstains from design and structure.

Pyola, which contains canola oil and pyrethrins, is persuading in killing aphids, squash bugs, and scarabs.

Other known garden pesticides are sabadilla, neem and pyrethrin.

Tomato leaf can likewise go about as bug sprinkle by smashing the leaves and eliminating the juice close by water and cornstarch. Utilize this depending upon the situation.

CHAPTER TWO

THE VARIOUS TYPES OF VERMIN CONTROL

Dispose of their food keep food set aside in fixed gatherings or the cooler; discard garbage, pieces and oil particularly from breaks and fissure. Remember pet food forgot about or opened sacks left in the pantry or carport. For a relentless pet food pervasion place pet food bowl in a bigger shallow dish load up with water to make a characteristic hindrance. Killing however much as could reasonably be expected eliminates the nuisance's food source. Dispose of their water search for areas of abundance dampness like under sinks, shower/shower regions, high temp water warmers, over-flooding at outside border, and cooling units re-direct or wipe out to eliminate irritation's water source. Drains holding decaying natural leaf matter ought to be cleaned consistently. Dispose of their homes-examine capacity regions at inside and outside and either place away from the construction, for example, kindling or spot in plastic sealed shut canisters to take out irritation's harborage regions. Recall this incorporates the carport and upper room particularly on the off chance that cardboard capacity boxes are being utilized. Plastic is suggested as cardboard is the ideal home since it very well may be a food source and a "nursery" for bothers. Dispose of branches and trim plants excessively near structure. Fend managed around 2 feet off to eliminate simple going from plant/tree to structure passage focuses. Dispose of passage focuses assess structure outside and seal up clear section focuses around electrical channels, pipes, windows and entryways. Froth sealant in a can is a fast as well as cheap fix. Weather conditions stripping at windows and entryways won't just keep out bothers however further develop energy productivity. Dispose of over the counter pesticides in the event that you are not getting results. Use pesticides astutely comprehend how they work and why. Know how to utilize them and what bothers they influence. Ineffectual utilization of pesticide isn't simply a misuse of cash however an ecological danger for your family and pets. It means a lot to know how to utilize the pesticide, where it tends to be utilized, how much and how frequently to utilize it. Over application is all around as terrible as under application. Applying some unacceptable items at some unacceptable regions will just objective the vermin to dissipate and increase. Dispose of unlicensed implement's who are "doing it as an afterthought" the risk is eventually not worth the reserve funds if any. The customer has no plan of action imagine a scenario where the implement is harmed on your property. Consider the possibility that misapplication of pesticide causes injury/harm to you or your neighbors or pets. Or then again more terrible yet is applying pesticide you can't see erroneously in your home? An authorized, guaranteed and reinforced state managed Bug Control supplier should meet thorough rules to get and keep up with their licenses. This is to safeguard the buyer. Realize your vermin control supplier and ensure they are without a doubt state authorized and guaranteed. Check whether they have a place with industry related associations and shopper insurance associations like the Better Business Department.

MOST NORMAL BUG CONTROL MISSTEPS

Buying over the counter showers and self-treating. Numerous supermarket items just don't give enduring advantages and at last reason more difficulty than they are worth. Assuming you as of now have an irritation control supplier ordinarily the shower you buy is a contact repellant that kills the nuisances you see however has no enduring lingering and really taints the expert items set up. Utilizing repellant showers cause a peculiarity called "sprouting" with numerous types of insects. The specialists are killed and don't get back to the settlement. The settlement will then, at that point, make more sovereigns and they will "bud" making more states! Bugs pervasions may briefly lessen however the hatchlings will before long incubate. Splashes for Blood sucker invasions wind up spreading the pervasion as they will keep away from the showered regions for a brief time frame. My idea would be on the off chance that you have an infrequent attacking irritation spritz it with window cleaning splash same outcome more affordable and most certainly less poisonous! On-going bug issues need proficient treatment.

Beginning a bug control administration while you see bothers and halting when you don't see bug. The vermin you don't see are not really gone - they are taken care of. Vermin will stay in the climate and will constantly be searching for food, water and harborage. The vermin control's supplier will likely control them in your current circumstance. Halting assistance since you don't see vermin will prompt irritation populaces gaining out of influence in the future. Reliable and standard bug control administration will break that cycle. Not knowing and understanding the Vermin Control supplier's treatment plan. Ensure you know and comprehend how your supplier is doing your administration. Seek clarification on pressing issues, really take a look at licenses, ask what they are treating your property with and why. Your Vermin Control supplier ought to have the option to give answers and ideas to your irritation control needs. "Green" items are routinely utilized in the business today to lessen natural effect. Figure out what items will work for your home. Assuming that your Vermin control supplier is by all accounts simply checking out your property figure out why-better specialists will constantly review before truly applying item. Advance additional about IPM rehearses from your supplier. In the event that they don't give data and treatment plans consolidating IPM Practices and "Green" items call an organization that can!

CHAPTER THREE

CULTIVATING AND NUISANCE CONTROL UNCOVERED

In spite of the fact that it appears to be somewhat simple to set up planting and vermin control, there are numerous things that you should think about first. As a matter of fact, a large number of the things that you'll learn about here are not examined frequently. Cultivating and bother control is essentially as old as horticulture. An industry's developing quickly. The nuisance control business has developed in excess of 50% over the most recent 5 years or somewhere in the vicinity, and cross country it has turned into a \$7 billion industry. With additional homes being inherent provincial regions the issue of irritation control has become more critical.

WHAT IS CULTIVATING AND IRRITATION CONTROL

It's fundamentally the decrease or annihilation of irritations. While primary irritation control is the control of family vermin and wood-obliterating nuisances and life forms or such different bugs which might attack families or designs, cultivating and bug control will in general be the control of irritations that are influencing your plants, yard as well as soil. That can at times pour out over into the house also however all around it's the nursery we're discussing here. To safeguard our developing regions as well as our wellbeing, legitimate planting and nuisance control is a need. It is frequently overlooked until bugs and their harm are found or it has insane. Well there are measures you can take to assist with annihilating the issue.

HOW WOULD WE CONTROL IRRITATIONS IN THE NURSERY

Many individuals see cultivating and bug control as a DIY work. Well that is all good to a limited extent. Cultivating irritation control resembles visiting the specialist: to recommend powerful treatment your doctor should accurately analyze the issue and decide the degree of the injury as well as the potential for additional injury. In overviews, it's been found that numerous householders try not to peruse the guidelines cautiously or want to change the directions 'since they feel they realize much improved'.

That prompts over-concentrated dosages of insect spray for instance which could be risky to your wellbeing and any guests. Obviously we are explicitly alluding to synthetics, as substance bother control is as yet the prevalent sort today. Nonetheless, all things considered, the drawn out impacts of synthetic compounds has prompted a restored interest in customary and natural vermin control towards the finish of the twentieth hundred years. For the individuals who don't Do-It-Yourself cultivating and bug control, there is the choice of month to month visits from your nearby organization. One benefit is that somebody ought to be taking a gander at your home and nursery for bug issues routinely. One inconvenience is that property holders demand that PCOs apply a compound treatment month to month regardless of whether there is a vermin issue. Current realities of pesticide use in the home and nursery are extremely astonishing:

- Every year 67 million pounds of pesticides are applied to yards.

- Rural yards and nurseries get far heavier pesticide applications per section of land than most agrarian regions.

Think before you shower a pesticide. You might kill the bugs that are assisting you with holding nuisances under wraps. This implies you should shower more from now on. Additionally, bugs benefit your nursery by pollinating your plants, helping them develop and proliferate. Try not to utilize industrious, expansive range, contact bug sprays like diazinon, malathion and carbaryl. These give just brief irritation control and are probably going to kill a greater amount of the regular foes than the vermin. At the point when their foes are gone, bother populaces might take off and turn out to be to a greater extent and issue as opposed to before they were showered.

Most buyers additionally don't understand how possibly destructive they can be:

- Pesticides are effortlessly followed inside
- An EPA concentrate on tracked down 23 pesticides in residue and air inside homes.

- Yard synthetics can hurt pets. Canine proprietors who utilize the herbicide 2, 4, D at least multiple times per season, twofold their canine's gamble of creating lymphoma. It's an enlightening shock isn't it? Will we extremely not be without these techniques for bother control?

CHAPTER FOUR

PLANTING AND REGULAR VERMIN CONTROL

We accept the coherent way to deal with planting and irritation control is to make equilibrium of creatures in your yard or nursery. Regular bug control is more affordable than purchasing and applying pesticides, and it's more secure for your nursery, normal untamed life and the climate. We should see a few clues and tips to assist you're planting and bug with controlling:

- Advantageous bugs that go after issue bugs are ready to move

- On the off chance that a plant, even a tree, has bug or infection issues consistently, now is the right time to supplant it with a more open minded assortment, or one more kind of plant that doesn't have these issues.

- By keeping nuisances from arriving at your plants, you can stay away from the harm they cause. Furthermore, in situations where you just see a couple of bugs, genuinely eliminating them can frequently monitor the issue. We should likewise take a gander at a few helpful bugs you need to empower in your nursery:

Bacillus thuringiensis (B.t.)

Undeniable hornet

Centipede

Damselfly

Ground creepy crawly

Bumble bee

Artisan honey bee

Parasitic wasp

Trooper insect

Yellow coat

Utilize these tips to make managing planting and nuisance control significantly more straightforward. Assuming that you follow the fundamentals you will practically take out your concern of nursery bugs until the end of time.

PROFITING FROM NATURAL NUISANCE CONTROL

Bug control is no simple assignment. In best case scenarios regular nuisances like bugs, rodents, and the like won't be in our living quarters by any means however can we just be look at things objectively for a moment, life isn't really great. When bugs figure out how to get into your house, it's difficult to make them disappear, and their presence could influence your wellbeing, your solace, and, surprisingly, your property! The more you leave the issue untreated, the more terrible it will be. One of the quickest methods for disposing of the little suckers is to shoot them with synthetics. Nonetheless, the simple methodology is presently leisurely being demonstrated to be a risky one research has shown that the utilization of compound specialists in pesticides as well as other man-made or engineered materials utilized for controlling bug can be as deadly to people for what it's worth to the critters you need to destroy. The perils are higher for kids as well as trained creatures, and on the off chance that you have either or both in your family, you would be advised to reconsider your choices or lament placing your friends and family in hurt. Fortunately, because of the progressions in current examination, non-poisonous and normally natural nuisance control techniques are presently generally accessible.

Natural vermin control techniques includes the utilization of regular instruments like normal predation, parasitism, and herbivore to control and annihilate bugs like bugs and bugs, and plant inconveniences like weeds and aphids. Natural bug control is one significant part of what is called coordinated bug the executives programs. Incorporated bother the executives is a characteristic way to deal with controlling bug which utilizes normal irritation foes to diminish the quantity of attacking nuisances with the dynamic assistance of human dispersion gradually. Parasitoids, hunters, and microbes, otherwise called organic log control specialists, are the normal adversaries of bug bothers.

Substance pesticides, as indicated by the Natural Insurance Organization, have been connected to instances of disease, nerve harm, and birth deserts among a heap of other unexpected issues. It is because of these perils that one ought to consider changing to natural nuisance control for of wiping out bugs. The cycle includes going after the nuisances in three stages. First: the joining of irritation anti-agents in the impacted region; second, the support of bug lessening bugs and different life forms, and in conclusion applying natural, at times home-prepared non-poisonous pesticides. Natural bug control brews are comprised of different combinations of solid smelling substances, scent atoms and gases in plants, cleanser, saponins or oils.

Rank substances like fish, garlic, or tomatoes can be utilized to repulse unsafe nuisances that might make harm plants. Cottonseed oils, mineral oils and other vegetable oils might be utilized to suffocate delicate bodied bothers. Heat as well as vapor from bean stew or lamp oil and salt is utilized to stop, consume, and kill bothers also.

These days, natural vermin control and its utilization for nearby bug the board are spearheading creative ways for less hurtful strategies for controlling irritation, and a large number of these neighborhood bother the executives procedures are straightforward and utilize. Utilizing traps is one strategy for overseeing nuisance that natural irritation control organizations are supporting however the actual thought is sufficiently straightforward. Traps intended to catch explicit sorts of bug irritations are presently generally accessible and are become more expense productive and successful. Neighborhood bug the executives is best done when one eliminates the nuisances from one region over a controlled and normal timeframe as opposed to out of nowhere clearing out entire populaces of both terrible and valuable creatures with a synthetic specialist. Presently when most awful comes to most terrible and you have no clue about how to deal with it any longer. The beneficial thing to do is to call your neighborhood bug the executive's administration. Without a doubt, there are bunches of capable bug the executives organizations in your space, you should simply to look and make a few inquiries.

THE END